Tight Hip Flexors

THE BENEFITS OF STRENGTHENING YOUR HIP FLEXORS: A COMPREHENSIVE GUIDE

Q. TITTERINGTON

Table of Contents

CHAPTER ONE

INTRODUCTION TO TIGHT HIP FLEXORS

Are you feeling tightness and pain in your hip area? In that case, you are not alone. Many individuals, from athletes to workplace workers, will experience tight hip flexors at some unspecified time in the future of their lives. In this blog post, we can delve into the subject of tight hip flexors, exploring the causes, signs and symptoms, and treatments. Whether or not you're an avid health enthusiast or clearly someone seeking to enhance your average well-being, expertise in the impact of tight hip flexors can be instrumental in attaining premier fitness. So, let's dive in and find out the bits and bobs of this commonplace difficulty that influences limitless people across the globe.

Are you experiencing pain or tightness in your hip region? In that case, you're no longer by yourself. Many individuals, from athletes to office employees, struggle with tight hip flexors. We will explore the subject of tight hip flexors and delve into the diverse reasons, symptoms, and potential solutions. Whether or not you are an avid runner searching for alleviation or, in reality, curious about this common issue, this introductory manual is right here to help you benefit from a higher expertise of tight hip flexors. Let's leap right in!

We're diving into the captivating world of tight hip flexors. Whether or not you're an athlete trying to enhance your performance, a workplace employee combating lower back pain, or certainly someone curious about the human body, this newsletter is for you. Tight hip flexors are a common difficulty that may affect humans of all ages and lifestyles. We will explore the causes of tight hip flexors, the capacity results, and, most importantly, sensible hints and sporting activities that will help you deal with this issue. So, get ready to free up the secrets and techniques of your hip flexors and find out the course toward multiplied mobility and typical well-being. Let's get started!

Where in we delve into a topic that influences many human beings: tight hip flexors. Whether you are an office employee sitting at a desk all day, an athlete pushing your body to its limits, or certainly someone who wants to improve flexibility and mobility, knowing the impact of tight hip flexors is prime. In this newsletter, we will explore the causes, signs and symptoms, and capacity answers for this not unusual difficulty. So whether or not you're experiencing discomfort or are genuinely curious about the topic, let's get started on this journey closer to unlocking the secrets and techniques of tight hip flexors.

Whether or not you are an athlete trying to enhance your overall performance, a health enthusiast aiming to optimize your workouts, or a genuinely curious person about the human frame, in this article we will discover the concept of tight hip flexors, their reasons, and their effect on our everyday lives.

Are you experiencing occasional hip pain or feeling tightness in your hip area? If so, you're no longer alone. Many people, irrespective of age or interest level, struggle with tight hip flexors. we can delve into the concern of tight hip flexors, exploring what they are, why they can emerge as tight, and the impact they are able to have on your ordinary well-being. Whether you are an athlete trying to enhance your performance or a person searching for relief from hip soreness, this newsletter is for you. So let's dive in and unravel the secrets of tight hip flexors.

BRIEFLY PROVIDE AN EXPLANATION FOR THE IMPORTANCE OF WHOLESOME HIP FLEXORS.

In our quest for normal health and well-being, we regularly forget the importance of maintaining wholesome hip flexors. Those muscles play an important function in our daily actions and can significantly affect our general bodily performance and quality of life. Whether or not you're an athlete, a fitness enthusiast, or, in reality, a person who wants to lead a lively and pain-free way of life, knowledge of the significance of healthy hip flexors is fundamental Join us as we delve into the sector of hip flexors and discover how their well-being can positively influence your physical fitness.

1. Beautify flexibility and variety of motion:

Wholesome hip flexors are responsible for permitting us to carry out a variety of actions, including walking, jogging, leaping, and even sitting. Those muscle groups allow us to move our legs and hips conveniently and manageably. While our hip flexor muscle tissues are tight or vulnerable, our flexibility and variety of movement can be significantly restricted. Through maintaining robust and flexible muscle tissue, we can revel in extra mobility, advanced athletic overall performance, and a reduced danger of injury.

2. Improve posture and stability:

The hip flexor muscle mass directly affects the alignment of our pelvis, backbone, and posture. While these muscles are susceptible or imbalanced, they could pull our pelvis forward, inflicting a posterior pelvic tilt. This misalignment can cause poor posture, decrease back pain, and improve strain on different surrounding muscle masses. By preserving healthy hip flexors, we can improve our posture, enhance center stability, and alleviate unnecessary strain on our frame, leading to better common body mechanics.

3. Alleviate or decrease backache:

Many individuals are afflicted by continual lower back pain, which may be attributed to tight hip flexor muscular tissues. While those muscles become tight or overactive, they are able to pull on the lower back, leading to pain. By strengthening and stretching the hip flexors, we will alleviate lower back pain and create a more fit spine.

4. Raise athletic performance:

Athletes of all degrees and sports depend on healthy hip flexors to enhance their performance. Whether or not you are a runner, bike owner, martial artist, or take part in some other recreation, having strong and bendy hip flexor muscle tissues can improve your pace, agility, and explosiveness. Sturdy hip flexors enable green stride duration, proper knee drive, and the most reliable hip extension, providing you with an aggressive edge in your chosen area.

5. Save you harm and imbalances:

Retaining healthy hip flexors plays an important role in injury prevention and maintaining overall muscle stability. Weak or tight hip flexors can disrupt the delicate balance between muscle mass, leading to compensatory actions and an expanded risk of injuries in other areas, including the knees or lower back. By incorporating ordinary hip flexor sports into your fitness routine, you may lessen the chance of imbalances, improve balance, and decrease the chance of injuries.

Our hip flexor muscle tissues are the powerhouse behind many crucial actions and sports in our everyday lives. By prioritizing the health and versatility of these muscle groups, we can release a myriad of benefits, from more suitable flexibility and range of motion to stepped-forward posture, decreased ache, and better athletic performance. Whether or not you are an athlete or a person looking for an energetic and pain-free lifestyle, do not underestimate the importance of healthy hip flexors. Invest time and effort into incorporating focused sporting activities and stretches into your routine.

SPOTLIGHT THE NOT-UNUSUAL TROUBLES RELATED TO TIGHT HIP FLEXORS.

Tight hip flexors are a tremendous problem that many humans won't even be aware of. Those muscle tissues, located inside the front of the hip, play an essential role in numerous moves, which include strolling, going for walks, or even sitting. However, while those muscles end up tight and rigid, it can lead to quite a number of troubles that can negatively impact your everyday life. In this blog post, we will highlight some of the commonplace issues associated with tight hip flexors and provide some hints on how to alleviate them.

1. Decrease lower back pain: one of the most common problems resulting from tight hip flexors is decreased back pain.

While the hip flexors are tight, they are able to pull on the lower back, causing pain and stiffness. This can be especially elaborate for those who spend lengthy hours sitting at a table or have a sedentary lifestyle. By releasing the anxiety inside the hip flexors, you can help relieve backaches, decrease back pain, and enhance your common posture.

2. Hip pain and pain: Tight hip flexors can also cause ache and discomfort at once within the hip area. This can make it tough to perform simple responsibilities, including walking or climbing stairs. In case you regularly experience hip pain, it is probably well worth considering whether or not your hip flexors are tight and in need of stretching and strengthening physical activities.

3. Restricted variety of motion: Another issue related to tight hip flexors is restricted variety of movement. When those muscles are tight, they are able to restrict actions within the hip joint, making it tough to perform physical games or participate in sports that require flexibility. This may be particularly irritating for athletes or folks who experience activities that include yoga or dancing. By using running to liberate the anxiety within the hip flexors, you could enhance your variety of motion and regain your potential to transport freely.

4. Terrible Posture: Tight hip flexors can contribute to bad posture, particularly in a circumstance known as anterior pelvic tilt. This takes place while the hip flexors pull the pelvis ahead, causing an exaggerated curvature in the lower back. Now, not only

can this result in lower back aches, but it could additionally affect the alignment of the whole spine. With the aid of addressing tight hip flexors, you can help correct your posture and alleviate related pain.

5. Reduced athletic performance: Athletes, in particular, may be significantly tormented by tight hip flexors. Those muscles are crucial for generating electricity and explosiveness in moves like sprinting, jumping, and kicking. When the hip flexors are tight, they can restrict the capacity to generate pressure efficaciously, resulting in reduced overall performance and an expanded chance of harm. Incorporating hip flexor stretches and physical games into your education can help improve athletic performance and prevent accidents.

Now that we've highlighted a number of the not-unusual problems related to tight hip flexors, it's vital to learn how to alleviate them. Stretching and strengthening exercises focused on the hip flexors can help release anxiety and enhance flexibility. Incorporating everyday movement breaks all through the day can also prevent the muscle tissues from becoming tight because of extended sitting. In case you are experiencing persistent soreness or pain related to tight hip flexors, it is advisable to consult with a healthcare expert or a certified health teacher who can offer personalized guidance and sporting activities tailored to your precise desires.

Tight hip flexors can result in more than a few issues, including lower back pain, hip ache, confined range of movement, bad posture, and reduced athletic overall performance. By understanding the common troubles related to tight hip flexors and taking proactive measures to deal with them, you could enhance your general well-being and quality of life. Don't allow tight hip flexors to maintain your return; begin incorporating hip flexor stretches and sporting events into your routine today!

CHAPTER TWO

EXPLAIN THE ANATOMY AND CHARACTERISTICS OF HIP FLEXOR MUSCLE TISSUE.

The hip flexor muscle groups are an essential organization of muscle mass placed within the front of your hip, accountable for the flexion of the hip joint. They play an essential role in diverse every-day activities, including walking, jogging, and even sitting down. Knowledge of the anatomy and features of those muscle groups allows you to better respect their significance and cope with them.

Anatomy of the Hip Flexor Muscles

The hip flexor muscle tissue encompasses a collection of muscle tissue referred to as the iliopsoas, which includes the psoas, which is the most important, and the iliacus. The psoas important originates from the lumbar backbone and runs down through the pelvis, attaching to the femur bone. The iliacus muscle originates from the iliac fossa, a part of the pelvis, and additionally attaches to the femur bone. Collectively, these two muscle groups work synergistically to perform hip flexion.

Characteristics of the hip flexor muscle tissue:

The number one characteristic of the hip flexor muscular tissues is to carry your thigh closer to your torso, which allows for moves like lifting your knee, bending ahead, or bringing your leg up at the same time as strolling or jogging. Those muscles are also concerned with maintaining a very good posture while standing or sitting upright.

IMPORTANCE OF PRESERVING HEALTHY HIP FLEXORS

Having sturdy and flexible hip flexor muscular tissues is critical for universal lower-body power and mobility. Neglecting their care can result in diverse troubles, including muscle imbalances, hip joint troubles, and even lower back pain. Sedentary lifestyles and extended sitting, which many of us are familiar with, can contribute to tightness and weak spots in the hip flexors.

Exercises to bolster and stretch the hip flexors:

To preserve healthy hip flexor muscle groups, incorporating stretching and strengthening sporting events into your daily routine may be beneficial. Here are some exercises to get you started:

1. Hip Flexor Stretch:

Kneel on one knee with the other leg bent in front of you.

Lean forward, preserving your back directly, till you sense a stretch within the front of your hip.

Preserve this role for 30 seconds and repeat on the alternative aspect.

2. Leg raises:

Lie flat on your back, along with your legs, immediately.

Lift one leg closer to your chest, keeping the knee straight, and slowly decrease the backtrack.

Repeat this motion 10–15 times on every leg.

3. Lunges:

Stand with one foot ahead and the alternative foot lower back.

Bend each knee, decreasing your frame until the returned knee is just above the floor.

Push through the front foot to go back to the beginning function.

Repeat this workout on every leg for 10–15 repetitions.

Don't forget to warm up before performing any sporting events and consult with a healthcare expert if you have any underlying situations or issues.

The hip flexor muscle tissue is a vital organization of muscles responsible for hip flexion and maintaining correct posture. Understanding their anatomy and features will help you respect their significance and take steps to keep them healthy. By incorporating exercises that stretch and fortify these muscle groups.

THE ROLE OF HIP FLEXORS IN THE FRAME'S MOTION

In terms of the body's movement, there's a group of muscle mass that frequently goes unnoticed but plays an important role in our daily activities. Those muscle groups are known as the hip flexors, and they are responsible for flexing the hip joint and permitting us to perform various actions, which include taking walks, strolling, or even sitting down.

The hip flexors are a collection of muscle tissue placed at the front of the hip, inclusive of the psoas essential, psoas minor, and iliacus muscle tissues. Those muscle groups work together to move the hip joint, permitting us to lift our legs and convey our knees toward our chest. This motion is essential for diverse sports that require decreased frame electricity and mobility.

One of the primary functions of the hip flexors is to help the leg move. While we walk or run, the hip flexors settle and pull the leg ahead, propelling us ahead. Without the hip flexors, we would not be able to circulate our legs correctly, and our ability to stroll or run could be significantly restrained.

Further to taking walks and strolling, the hip flexors additionally play a considerable role in other activities consisting of cycling, jumping, and kicking. Those muscular tissues are responsible for producing strength and pressure, permitting us to interact in sports and activities that require explosive movements. Sturdy hip flexors are essential for athletes and those who take part in activities that require short and effective movements.

Furthermore, the hip flexors also play an important function in maintaining proper posture. While the hip flexors are tight or weak, they can pull the pelvis ahead, inflicting an anterior pelvic tilt. This misalignment can result in lower back pain, hip ache, or even knee ache. Consequently, it's far more important to keep the hip flexors flexible and strong to maintain the right posture and avoid any soreness or pain.

Sadly, due to our sedentary existence and prolonged sitting, many people have tight hip flexors. Sitting for extended periods can cause the hip flexors to become shortened and tight, leading to terrible posture and confined mobility. Therefore, it's vital to incorporate hip flexor stretches and exercises into our day-to-day routine to maintain flexibility and save you any capacity troubles.

A few effective hip flexor stretches include the kneeling hip flexor stretch, the status hip flexor stretch, and the butterfly stretch. These stretches target the hip flexors, helping to lengthen and release any tension in these muscle groups. Moreover, strengthening sporting events including leg increases, lunges, and squats can also improve the strength and versatility of the hip flexors.

The hip flexors play a large role in the frame's movement, from walking and jogging to jumping and kicking. Those muscular tissues are responsible for flexing the hip joint and generating strength and pressure. It's crucial to preserve the hip flexors' flexibility and strength through ordinary stretching and strengthening sporting events to maintain proper posture, prevent discomfort, and enhance typical mobility. So, the next time you lace up your shoes for a run or get ready for exercise, consider the importance of your hip flexors and give them the attention they deserve.

CHAPTER THREE

PROVIDE EXAMPLES OF SPORTS THAT MAY PRESSURE THE HIP FLEXORS.

Hip flexors play a crucial function in our everyday movements, allowing us to stroll, run, and perform diverse exercises. But those muscle tissues can, on occasion, turn out to be strained, leading to pain, constrained mobility, and even injury. In this article, we can discover seven common activities that may stress your hip flexors and offer recommendations on how to prevent such injuries. Whether or not you're an athlete, a fitness fanatic, or sincerely seeking to preserve a wholesome lifestyle, understanding these sports will assist you in protecting your hip flexors and living an active life pain-free.

1. Prolonged sitting:

Sitting for prolonged periods can cause your hip flexor muscular tissues to shorten and tighten. This could lead to imbalances in your hip joint, resulting in strain and discomfort. If you have a desk task or spend extended hours sitting, it's critical to take everyday breaks and carry out hip flexor stretches to counteract the results of extended sitting.

2. Excessive-depth physical activities:
Activities that involve repetitive hip flexion, along with high-intensity cardio language education (HIIT) sporting activities, sprinting, or kickboxing, can place massive strain on the hip flexor muscle tissue. While those exercises are awesome for cardiovascular fitness, it's essential to ensure the right heat-up, stretching, and slow progression to avoid overloading the hip flexors.

3. Long-distance jogging:

Runners, mainly the ones training for marathons or participating in lengthy-distance walking, often experience hip flexor strain due to the repetitive actions. To keep from straining your hip flexors, it's vital to incorporate cross-training exercises, strength education, and regular stretching routines into your jogging regimen.

4. Biking:

Cycling is an amazing low-impact workout for cardiovascular fitness and leg power. However, the repetitive movement of pedaling can cause hip flexor strain if not executed with proper form or with enough warm-up and stretching. Carrying out hip flexor stretches earlier and after cycling can help prevent accidents and preserve flexibility.

5. Overhead Lifting:

Weightlifting exercises that contain overhead movements, such as overhead presses or snatches, can strain the hip flexor muscle tissue. These moves require sizeable balance and mobility within the hip joint, making it vital to ensure the right approach, center engagement, and hip flexibility to save you pressure.

6. Excessive Sitting in a Chair with Legs Striking:

Sitting in a chair with your legs unsupported for lengthy durations can place unnecessary strain on your hip flexors, leading to pain and tightness. To minimize pressure, make certain you've got proper support in your feet and keep in mind using a footrest. Regularly changing your sitting position and performing hip flexor stretches during breaks is likewise beneficial.

7. Insufficient heat-up and stretching:

No matter what hobby you have, neglecting proper warm-up and stretching can greatly increase the danger of hip flexor lines. Heat-united states need to encompass dynamic actions that focus on the hip flexors, along with leg swings or lunges, to boost blood flow and put together the muscle groups for the activity. Submit-activity stretching ought to focus on lengthening and liberating tension within the hip flexors.

Knowledge of the sports that could stress your hip flexors is essential to preventing accidents and maintaining your general well-being. Whether or not you are an avid athlete, fitness enthusiast, or someone who sits for lengthy hours, incorporating effective warm-up exercises, the right form, and ordinary hip flexor stretching into your routine will help protect your hip flexors and improve your average mobility. Don't forget, a little greater care can go a long way in preserving your hip flexors' health and making them pain-free.

CHAPTER FOUR

SYMPTOMS OF TIGHT HIP FLEXORS

Are you experiencing pain in your hips? It can be a sign of tight hip flexors. Hip flexors are a group of muscle tissues that can help you raise your knees and bend at the waist. They play a crucial role in regular movements, which include walking, jogging, and even sitting. But when these muscle groups turn out to be tight and rigid, it can cause signs that affect your day-to-day lifestyle. We will explore the symptoms and signs of tight hip flexors, as well as the reasons for them and remedy alternatives.

1. Lower lower back ache: Tight hip flexors can cause improved strain at the lower back, leading to pain and soreness. That is due to the fact that when the hip flexor

muscles are tight, they can pull at the pelvis, causing it to tilt ahead and creating an immoderate curve in the lower back. This could result in persistent lower back pain that will get worse with extended sitting or sports that contain hip flexion.

2. Hip ache: another not unusual symptom of tight hip flexors is an ache or pain in the hip joints. Tight muscle tissues can cause impingement or compression of systems within the hip joint, leading to pain in the front of the hip or deep in the joint itself. This could make sports like walking, squatting, or mountain climbing uncomfortable.

3. Decreased variety of motion: while your hip flexor muscle tissues are tight, they are able to restrict your hip's range of movement. This can make it hard to perform actions that require hip extension,

such as kicking, lunging, or maybe standing up directly. You may sense stiffness or tightness in the front of your hips, restricting your ability to transport freely.

4. Bad posture: Tight hip flexors can contribute to negative posture, in particular a forward pelvic tilt. While the hip flexors are tight, they could pull the pelvis forward, causing an exaggerated curve in the lower back and a sticking abdomen. This will lead to an imbalanced posture, putting strain on other muscle groups and doubtless leading to muscle imbalances and pain in other regions of the body.

5. Problem in center activation: The hip flexors are related to the center muscle mass, and while they may be tight, they are able to inhibit right center activation. This will have an effect on your stability

and electricity, making it harder to interact with your stomach muscle groups and preserve a robust middle. Weak middle muscular tissues can lead to a selection of troubles, including decreased return pain and reduced athletic overall performance.

Now that we've explored the signs and symptoms of tight hip flexors, let's discuss some possible causes and treatment alternatives. One not unusual reason for tight hip flexors is prolonged sitting, as this position maintains the hip flexors in a shortened position for prolonged durations. Different elements, together with overuse, muscle imbalances, and insufficient stretching, can also contribute to tightness in the hip flexor muscle tissues.

Fortunately, there are several methods to relieve tight hip flexors and decrease related signs. First and foremost, regular stretching and flexibility sports events that target the hip flexors can assist in prolonging and releasing anxiety in this muscle tissue. Incorporating hip mobility exercises into your health routine can also improve flexibility and variety of movement.

Similarly to stretching and mobility sports, strengthening sporting activities for the glutes and center can help to rebalance the muscle tissue across the hips, decreasing the stress on the hip flexors. This can consist of sporting activities such as squats, lunges, bridges, and planks.

In case your signs persist or worsen, it's always really useful to visit a healthcare expert. They can offer a thorough assessment, diagnose the underlying purpose of your tight hip flexors, and suggest appropriate remedy options, including physical remedies or other interventions.

Tight hip flexors can cause a number of symptoms that may impact your day-to-day lifestyle and normal well-being. With the aid of knowledge of the signs and symptoms of tight hip flexors, you could take proactive steps to address the problem and search for an appropriate remedy. Bear in mind to prioritize regular stretching, mobility sports, and energy schooling, and don't hesitate to look for expert guidance if desired. Take care of your hip flexors, and they will contend with you!

EXPLAIN HOW TIGHT HIP FLEXORS CAN HAVE AN EFFECT ON EVERYDAY SPORTS AND NORMAL POSTURE.

Do you ever find yourself experiencing soreness or pain in your lower back or hips? Have you ever wondered why certain day-to-day sports seem more difficult than they need to be? The solution may lie in your hip flexors. Many of us are ignorant of the impact tight hip flexors may have on our day-to-day lives and basic posture. We will delve into the intriguing world of hip flexors, exploring how their tightness can have an effect on your every-day sports and posture and what you can do to locate relief.

Before we delve deeper, it's essential to understand what hip flexors are and their function in our body. Hip flexors are a collection of muscle tissue located on the front of your hips, inclusive of the psoas foremost, iliacus, and rectus femoris. Those muscle masses play a critical role in permitting motion in the hip joint, which includes walking, running, and even sitting. While those muscular tissues are functioning optimally, they provide balance and flexibility to assist your body's actions. But once they become tight, a myriad of problems can arise.

The impact on every-day activities:

1. Taking walks and going for walks:

Tight hip flexors can drastically affect your gait and stride length, making walking or strolling more exhausting. Those muscles play a vital function in lifting your leg ahead at some point in each step. While they're tight, they restrict this movement, leading to a shortened stride and increased effort during those sports.

2. Sitting:

In the present-day sedentary way of life, sitting for prolonged intervals has become inevitable. Unfortunately, this will exacerbate the problem of tight hip flexors. When you take a seat, your hip flexors stay in a shortened position for prolonged intervals, causing them to end up chronically tight. This will result in discomfort, stiffness, and even an ache in the hips and lower back.

3. Stability and balance:

Tight hip flexors can compromise your balance and stability, affecting your capacity to carry out every-day sports that require coordination. Whether it is climbing stairs, bending down to pick something up, or reaching for gadgets, having tight hip flexors could make these actions more challenging and increase the chance of falls or injuries.

THE IMPACT ON POSTURE

1. Anterior Pelvic Tilt:

One of the most common postural issues associated with tight hip flexors is anterior pelvic tilt. This occurs when the hip flexors and lower back muscles turn out to be imbalanced, causing the pelvis to tilt forward. As an end result, you can expect an exaggerated curve to your lower back, a sticking stomach, and a standard misalignment of the backbone. This posture no longer only impacts your look but can also cause back pain, hip pain, and reduced core balance.

2. Rounded shoulders:

Tight hip flexors cannot directly contribute to poor top-frame posture, in particular in the shoulders. While the hip flexors are tight, they could tilt the pelvis forward, which in turn causes the top frame to lean backward. This misalignment can cause rounded shoulders, a hunched, higher back, or even neck soreness.

LOCATING COMFORT AND ENHANCING POSTURE:

1. Stretching and mobility sports activities: Incorporate ordinary stretching and mobility exercises, particularly those targeted at the hip flexors, to help alleviate tightness. Exercises like the kneeling hip flexor stretch, lunges, and yoga poses including the pigeon pose may be beneficial in lengthening these muscle groups and restoring flexibility.

2. Core Strengthening:

Engaging in core-strengthening sporting events can help rebalance the muscle mass surrounding the hip flexors. Strong belly muscle mass and a stable middle can offer aid to the pelvis and promote higher posture.

3. Posture awareness:

Practice conscious posture in the course of the day, taking note of how you sit, stand, and circulate. Make sure that your hips continue to be neutral and your spine is aligned, avoiding immoderate slumping or arching.

The effect of tight hip flexors on your daily sports and standard posture cannot be underestimated. From hindered mobility to postural imbalances, those muscle tissues can cause soreness and affect your ordinary well-being.

Do you frequently revel in tightness and discomfort in your hip area? If so, you may be dealing with tight hip flexors. This common difficulty influences many humans and might lead to numerous headaches if left unattended. We are able to explore the reasons for tight hip flexors, dropping light on the hidden culprits in the back of your soreness. Whether you are an athlete, a desk employee, or, in reality, someone seeking out solutions, this information is relevant to you

So, let's dive in!

1. Extended Sitting: One of the foremost causes of tight hip flexors is spending prolonged intervals of time in a seated position. Whether or not it's due to office work, using a computer, or watching TV,

sitting for long hours can cause shortening and tightening of the hip flexor muscles. This will result in reduced mobility and versatility, leading to soreness and aches.

2. Loss of bodily hobby: if you lead a sedentary way of life or do not interact in everyday exercise, your hip flexor muscle mass may additionally emerge as weak and tight. While those muscles are not stretched and reinforced frequently, they are able to lose their flexibility and come to be at risk of tightness and discomfort. Incorporating physical games that focus on the hip flexors, which include lunges or yoga poses, can help alleviate this issue.

3. Overuse and repetitive movements: positive sports or sports activities that involve repetitive hip flexor movements can contribute to tightness. Jogging, cycling, and kicking sports are examples of

activities that could put stress on these muscle groups and lead to tightness over the years. It's essential to stabilize your workout routine and include stretching and restoration techniques to avoid overuse injuries and maintain the most fulfilling hip flexibility.

4. Muscle Imbalances: Imbalances among the hip flexor muscle tissues and the opposing muscles, which include the glutes and hamstrings, can also contribute to tightness. While one muscle is more potent or tighter than the other, it can create an imbalance inside the hip joint, leading to discomfort and a restricted range of movement. Strengthening and stretching during sporting activities that target both the hip flexors and the opposing muscle tissue are essential to preserving balance and preventing tightness.

5. Pressure and emotional tension: it can come as a wonder, but strain and emotional anxiety can occur physically within the frame, such as the hip flexors. While we revel in pressure, our muscle mass tends to increase, and if we always hold tension in our hip flexors, it can result in tightness and pain. Incorporating pressure-lowering practices, which include meditation or deep respiratory sporting activities, can help relax the frame and alleviate tension in the hip flexor muscles.

Now that we have explored the diverse reasons for tight hip flexors, it is critical to recognize that everybody's scenario is particular. It is advisable to seek advice from a healthcare professional or a certified health teacher who can check your specific circumstances and provide personalized guidance. They are able to recommend appropriate sporting events, stretches, and way of life changes tailored to your desires. Tight hip flexors can have an effect on humans from all walks of life. Whether it is because of prolonged sitting, loss of physical interest, overuse, muscle imbalances, or stress, identifying the causes of your discomfort is step one towards locating alleviation. Through incorporating focused sporting activities, stretching workouts, and lifestyle modifications, you can gradually release tension and improve the ability of your hip flexors. Bear in mind that taking care of your frame is a non-stop adventure, and with the proper approach, you may regain consolation and mobility in your hips.

CHAPTER FIVE

THE IMPORTANCE OF STRETCHING

Where time is a treasured commodity, it is easy to overlook the simple act of stretching. However, incorporating stretching sporting activities into your everyday routine can have several benefits for your universal fitness and well-being. Whether you are a fitness enthusiast or a person who spends the majority of their day sitting at a desk, stretching should not be underestimated.

Why stretch subjects?

1. Stepped forward Flexibility: one of the most obvious benefits of stretching is more desirable flexibility. Regular stretching increases the range of motion in your joints and muscle mass, allowing you to move more freely. This could be especially useful

for athletes or those engaged in physical sports, as it is able to improve performance and decrease the threat of injuries.

2. Decreased muscle tension: Sitting for lengthy intervals or conducting repetitive activities can result in muscle tightness and tension. Stretching enables you to relieve this tension by relaxing the muscle mass and increasing blood flow. It may also relieve muscle discomfort after exercising, decreasing the probability of post-exercising discomfort.

3. More advantageous posture: Spending hours hunched over a display screen or sitting in mistaken positions can negatively affect your posture. Normal stretching can help counterbalance those outcomes by lengthening tight muscle groups and restoring proper alignment. By improving your posture, you may now not only look

more assured but also lessen the danger of developing musculoskeletal problems in the long run.

4. Strain remedy: Stretching isn't always just beneficial for your bodily well-being but also for your mental health. Conducting stretching physical games can help launch anxiety and decrease pressure stages. The rhythmic movements and consciousness required through stretching will have a calming impact on the mind, promoting relaxation and mindfulness.

5. Injury Prevention: whether you are an athlete or just going about your everyday activities, the hazard of damage is continually present. By incorporating stretching into your routine, you could appreciably lessen the likelihood of strains, sprains, and other not unusual accidents. Stretching allows you to heat up the

muscle tissues, grow their elasticity, and enhance their resilience, making them much less liable to harm at some point of physical interest.

6. Progressed move: Stretching stimulates blood to flow with the flow to the muscle mass, which may have a high-quality effect on the overall stream. Better blood circulation means extra oxygen and nutrients reach your muscles, aiding in their restoration and selling their most excellent characteristic. Additionally, stepped-forward flow can help lessen muscle cramps and improve typical cardiovascular fitness.

INCORPORATING STRETCHING INTO YOUR HABITUAL

Now that you understand the importance of stretching, you may be thinking about how to incorporate it into your day-to-day routine. Don't forget the subsequent suggestions:

1. Heat up: before engaging in any stretching sporting events, it's crucial to heat up your muscle tissues with a few mild cardio activities, such as walking or jogging. This enables you to put together your frame for stretching and reduces the threat of damage.

2. Stretch all important muscle groups: focus on stretching all essential muscle groups, inclusive of your neck, shoulders, back, chest, arms, hips, legs, and calves. Keep every stretch for 15–30 seconds

without bouncing, and repeat each stretch 2-3 times.

3. Stretching strategies: there are various stretching strategies to choose from, including static stretching, dynamic stretching, and proprioceptive neuromuscular facilitation (PNF) stretching. Experiment with extraordinary strategies to find what works well for you.

4. Make it a habit: Consistency is fundamental on the subject of stretching. goal is to stretch at least 3-5 times per week, if not each day. You could incorporate stretching into your warm-up and cool-down routines, as well as at some point during breaks throughout the day.

Consider constantly listening to your body and staying away from overstretching or stretching injured muscle mass. If you have any underlying clinical situations or worries, visit a healthcare expert before starting any new stretching routine.

Incorporating stretching into your everyday routine is an easy and effective way to improve your general health and well-being. From elevated flexibility to reduced muscle tension and strain relief, the advantages of stretching are extensive. So, whether you're an athlete, a hectic professional, or someone seeking to beautify their life, do not underestimate the importance of stretching. Take a couple of minutes each day to stretch, and you'll reap the rewards of a more flexible, comfortable, and healthy body.

STRENGTHENING PHYSICAL GAMES FOR HIP FLEXORS

Our hip flexors are an important group of muscle tissues that play a significant role in our daily sports, from strolling and jogging to sitting and standing. However, due to the sedentary nature of current lifestyles, many humans suffer from weak hip flexors, leading to various problems consisting of lower back aches, negative posture, and confined mobility. We will discover some powerful strengthening sporting events for hip flexors that allow you to liberate your complete potential and lead a more fit and active lifestyle.

1. Leg raises:

Leg increases are an easy but powerful exercise that targets the hip flexor muscle mass. To perform this workout, lie flat on your lower back with your legs extended. Slowly lift one leg off the ground, retaining it immediately, until it reaches a 45-degree angle with the ground. Maintain it Maintain it for some seconds, then lower it and backtrack. Repeat with the other leg Intention for 10–15 repetitions on every aspect, steadily growing as your energy improves.

2. Lunges:

Lunges are a fantastic compound workout that engages more than one muscle group, which includes the hip flexors. Begin by standing with your feet shoulder-width apart. Leap forward with one leg, bending your knee until it forms a 90-degree angle. Make certain your front knee does not expand past your toes. Thrust back as much as in the beginning position and repeat with the alternative leg. Perform

10–15 lunges on every leg, gradually increasing the intensity as you progress.

3. Seated knee raises:

This exercise is ideal for strengthening the hip flexors even while sitting. Take a seat on the threshold of a strong chair with your feet flat on the floor. Slowly raise one knee closer to your chest, preserving your lower back directly. Keep it for a few seconds, then decrease it and backpedal. Repeat with the alternative knee. Purposefully perform 10–15 repetitions on each side, gradually increasing the problem by conserving weight for your thigh.

4. Mountain climbers:

Mountain climbers are a dynamic workout that no longer only strengthens your hip flexors but also affords top-notch cardiovascular exercise. Start in a push-up position, with your arms immediately underneath your shoulders and your body in a straight line. Deliver one knee closer to your chest, then quickly transfer your legs, mimicking a jogging motion. Continue alternating legs for 30–60 seconds, or as long as you can preserve your right form.

5. Bridge Pose:

The bridge pose is a notable workout because it concentrates on the entire hip area, such as the hip flexors. Lie flat on your back with your knees bent and your feet flat on the floor. Slowly carry your hips off the floor, squeezing your glutes and your core. Hold this position for a few seconds, then lower your hips back. goal for 10–15 repetitions, steadily increasing the length of each keep.

Strengthening your hip flexors is crucial for retaining average stability, posture, and mobility. By incorporating these sporting activities into your fitness routine, you may alleviate soreness, reduce the risk of harm, and unlock your complete ability. Don't forget to begin slowly and gradually increase the depth as your electricity improves. If you experience any aches or pains, discuss them with a healthcare expert. Permit us to strengthen the hip flexors and embody a healthier, more active way of life!

LIFESTYLE ADJUSTMENTS TO PREVENT TIGHT HIP FLEXORS

Are you tired of handling tight hip flexors? Those muscular tissues play a crucial role in our regular movements, and once they become tight, they are able to cause pain and restrain mobility. The good news is that there are lifestyle adjustments you can make to prevent and alleviate this common problem. We are able to explore a few powerful strategies that each person can implement to keep their hip flexors healthy and bent.

1. Stretch regularly:

One of the handiest and simplest approaches to preventing tight hip flexors is through regular stretching. Include particular hip flexor stretches into your day-to-day routine to keep those muscles supple and flexible. A few famous stretches include the kneeling hip flexor stretch, the butterfly stretch, and the pigeon pose. Make certain to maintain every stretch for at least 30 seconds to permit the muscular tissues to correctly elongate.

2. Workout and enhance:

In addition to stretching, it's essential to exercise and reinforce your hip flexors. Have interaction in sports that focus on those muscle tissues, such as walking, cycling, and swimming. Additionally, attempt sporting activities like leg lifts, bridges, and lunges that especially target the hip flexor muscle mass. Constructing power in this vicinity can help you save tightness and improve average hip mobility.

3. Take common breaks:

Sitting for extended intervals can contribute to tight hip flexors. Whether or not you have a desk or spend a variety of time using it, it is crucial to take frequent breaks to arise, stretch, and stroll around. Set a timer to remind yourself to rise and move each hour. These brief breaks will help prevent your hip flexors from becoming stiff and tight due to extended sitting.

4. Maintain proper posture.

Poor posture can place extra strain on your hip flexor muscular tissues, leading to tightness and discomfort. Practice keeping a suitable posture for the duration of the day, whether you're sitting, standing, or walking. Preserve your shoulders, engage your core muscle mass, and align your spine nicely. By doing so, you could alleviate needless strain in your hip flexors and promote better average body alignment.

5. Mind your exercise form:

While conducting bodily activities or power-training sports, pay close attention to your form. Flawed form or method can place excessive stress on your hip flexors, leading to tightness and muscle damage. are seeking guidance from a certified fitness professional to ensure you are performing exercises correctly and using the right body mechanics.

6. Live hydrated:

Trust it or not, hydration can play a role in preserving the power of your muscle tissues, including your hip flexors. Make sure to drink enough water at some point in the day to keep your muscle groups properly hydrated. Dehydration can result in muscle tightness and cramping, so it is vital to stay hydrated to support standard muscle health.

7. Exercise strain control:

Pressure can cause anxiety within the body, along with the hip flexors. Include pressure control techniques into your daily routine, consisting of meditation, deep respiratory physical games, or yoga. By lowering stress levels, you can help relieve tightness in your hip flexors and promote rest throughout your whole body.

Keep in mind that stopping tight hip flexors is all about retaining a healthy way of life and incorporating mindful behavior into your ordinary routine. By stretching regularly, working out and strengthening, taking breaks, retaining the right posture, minding your exercise form, staying hydrated, and coping with pressure, you may keep your hip flexors glad and bendy.

If you're already experiencing tightness or discomfort in your hip flexors, it is essential to pay attention to your body and seek professional recommendations. A healthcare professional or a qualified physical therapist can provide guidance and personalized suggestions to help you cope with any current troubles and prevent additional discomfort.

By imposing these lifestyle modifications, you can keep your hip flexors in optimal condition, allowing you to travel without problems and in comfort. Take care of your frame, prioritize your hip flexor health, and enjoy the blessings of a pain-free and energetic lifestyle.

PREVENTING FUTURE TIGHTNESS

All of us experience tightness in our bodies every so often. Whether or not it's the stiffness in our muscles after a long day of labor or the tension in our shoulders due to stress, tightness may have a vast impact on our basic well-being. However, there are numerous methods to prevent and alleviate tightness before it becomes a habitual problem. We will explore powerful strategies and practices that allow you to maintain a more fit and cozy frame.

1. Incorporate stretching into your routine: Normal stretching is critical for preserving your muscles' flexibility and stopping tightness. Make it an addiction to dedicate a couple of minutes each day to stretching your primary muscle groups, which include your neck, shoulders, legs, and arms.

Incorporating stretching physical activities into your everyday routine will help improve your flexibility, grow your blood stream, and decrease the risk of muscle imbalances due to tightness.

2. Live energetically:

Physical interest is important for stopping tightness and maintaining normal fitness. Engaging in regular workouts now not only facilitates strengthening your muscular tissues but also improves flexibility and mobility. Recall incorporating activities like yoga, Pilates, or maybe an easy, brisk stroll into your day-to-day routine. Locating a pastime that you enjoy will not only assist in reducing your tightness but also contribute to a more fit lifestyle.

3. Exercise an exact posture:

Preserving excellent posture is frequently left out, but it plays an enormous role in preventing tightness. Poor posture can lead to muscle imbalances and stress in certain areas of your body, resulting in tightness and discomfort. Be aware of your posture throughout the day, whether you are sitting at a table or standing. Make certain that your backbone is aligned, your shoulders are aligned, and your head is lifted. Incorporating easy posture exercises and ergonomic changes for your workspace can also help alleviate future tightness.

4. Control strain:

Stress is not an unusual contributor to tightness in the body. When we're stressed, our muscle tissues tend to tighten up, leading to discomfort and tightness. Finding powerful stress control strategies along with meditation, deep respiratory physical activities, or sports you enjoy can help reduce stress levels and prevent destiny tightness. Prioritize self-care and find time for rest to promote normal well-being.

5. Live Hydrated:

Hydration performs a significant function in stopping muscle tightness. Dehydration can cause muscle cramps and stiffness, making it important to drink a sufficient quantity of water at some point in the day. Intentionally drink at least 8 glasses of water a day, and remember to stay hydrated before, during, and after workout classes. Additionally, incorporating hydrating ingredients like fruits and veggies into your diet can also contribute to universal hydration.

6. Get regular massages.

Normal massages may be a splendid way to prevent and alleviate destiny tightness. Massage therapy helps to loosen up muscles, improve blood flow, and release anxiety. Don't forget to schedule regular rubdown appointments to get the benefits of skilled hands and centered techniques that specifically cope with regions vulnerable to tightness.

Stopping future tightness is essential for maintaining a healthier and more relaxed frame. By incorporating stretching, staying energetic, working towards accurate posture, dealing with pressure, staying hydrated, and getting everyday massages, you may drastically lessen the probability of experiencing tightness in your muscle mass and joints. Don't forget, prevention is always better than cure in relation to keeping your body flexible, cellular, and ache-free. Take charge of your well-being and implement those strategies into your day-to-day routine to enjoy a more cozy and colorful existence.

On the subject of our universal fitness and well-being, we frequently neglect the importance of having flexible hips. Tight hip flexors, a not uncommon issue faced by many individuals, can lead to numerous discomforts and obstacles in daily life. But knowing the reasons and answers for tight hip flexors will assist you in finding the relief you want to live your existence to the fullest.

We have explored the subject of tight hip flexors and their impact on our bodies. We have delved into the reasons for tight hip flexors, which include prolonged sitting, loss of exercise, and terrible posture. Those factors can contribute to a shortening of the hip flexor muscle mass, leading to tightness and discomfort.

One of the most beneficial effects of tight hip flexors is a restricted range of movement. This will have an effect on numerous sports consisting of taking walks, running, or even sitting easily. It could additionally cause decreased back pain, hip pain, or even knee pain. Additionally, tight hip flexors can negatively affect your posture because the pelvis tilts ahead, causing an imbalance in your frame's alignment.

Thankfully, there are numerous approaches to coping with tight hip flexors and discovering the comfort you want. Ordinary stretching sports, in particular those focused on the hip flexor muscular tissues, can help lengthen and unfasten them. Incorporating sporting activities, which include lunges, hip openers, and yoga poses like the pigeon pose, into your routine may be extraordinarily useful. Moreover, it is essential to address the underlying reasons for tight hip flexors. If you have a sedentary lifestyle or spend a large amount of time sitting, take ordinary breaks to stretch and flow. Carrying out a regular workout, together with walking, running, or biking, can also help prevent and alleviate tight hip flexors.

Maintaining excellent posture at some point in the day is another important issue to keep in mind. Understand your sitting and standing posture, ensuring that your back is straight and your shoulders are comfortable. Investing in an ergonomic chair or using a cushion to help your lower back can also make a big difference.

Moreover, searching for expert assistance from a physical therapist or a chiropractor can provide you with personalized guidance and treatment alternatives. They can carry out unique assessments and provide exercises tailored to your individual wishes, helping you obtain excellent hip flexibility and overall well-being.

Tight hip flexors may be an unusual and uncomfortable issue for many individuals. However, by understanding the reasons, imposing stretching physical games, addressing underlying factors, and seeking expert assistance when desired, you can find relief and improve your pleasant lifestyle. Do not let tight hip flexors preserve you again to any extent; take the essential steps to regain your flexibility and maintain a pain-free, active lifestyle.

THE END

www.ingramcontent.com/pod-product-compliance
Lightning Source LLC
Chambersburg PA
CBHW050745260726
48661CB00001B/422